FEELING FIT

PARTICIPANT GUIDE

Linda Sorrells, MS, MA
Merry Anne Schmied, MS
Illinois State University

Life Enhancement Publications
Champaign, Illinois

Library of Congress Cataloging-in-Publication Data

Sorrells, Linda, 1938-
    Feeling fit: participant guide/Linda Sorrells, Merry Anne
Schmied.
        p.   cm.
    ISBN 0-87322-915-0.   ISBN 0-87322-916-9 (package)
    1. Health behavior.   2. Physical fitness.   3. Health.
  I. Schmied, Merry Anne, 1948-   . II. Title.
RA776.9.S67   1988
613—dc19   87-31117
                                                           CIP

Developmental Editor: Sue Wilmoth, PhD
Production Director: Ernie Noa
Projects Manager: Lezli Harris
Copy Editor: Peter Nelson
Assistant Editor: Julie Anderson
Typesetter: Yvonne Winsor
Text Design: Keith Blomberg
Text Layout: Denise Mueller
Printed By: Versa Press

ISBN: 0-87322-915-0
        0-87322-916-9 (Pkg.)

Feeling Fit videos were produced at Media Services Television, Illinois State University
under the direction of John Tannura.

Printed in the United States of America

10 9 8 7 6 5 4 3 2 1

Life Enhancement Publications
A Division of Human Kinetics Publishers, Inc.
Box 5076, Champaign, IL 61820

Contents

Preface

How happy are you with your current lifestyle? Would you make any changes? When your alarm rang this morning, was your first thought "forget it"? Did you avoid the scale and the full-length mirror? Were you thoroughly convinced you had to go on a diet, but then ate the last two doughnuts for breakfast? When you left the house, were you disgruntled with yourself, the weather, and the state of the world?

If you answered yes to two or three of these questions, you are one of the many people we are trying to reach through the Feeling Fit series. *Feeling Fit* is about YOU. It's about your wellness and ability to control your life. Wellness is a way of life involving self-acceptance and being responsible for your well-being. The choice to move to a higher level of wellness is yours.

This participant guide is designed to help you assess many facets of your lifestyle. You'll get chances to assess your level of stress, your diet, your physical fitness, and much more. Each lesson in the guide begins with an overview of information on its topic. Next, the "Video Connections" section will help you make important applications to your lifestyle from what you saw and heard on the screen. Informative "Healthy Highlights" have been extracted from the presentation. One of the most enjoyable portions of the lesson is the "Self-Assessment" section. This will give you the opportunity to see how you currently lead your lifestyle, which is important to understand before deciding which future directions to pursue. The "Prevention/ Promotion" section will provide you with insight into whether you prevent or promote wellness. "Well(ness) Worth Remembering" consists of summary points that you may want to keep for future use.

Taking an honest look at yourself is never easy but can be highly rewarding; try to approach these programs with as much honesty as you can. Don't be afraid to be yourself or to make decisions that can lead you to a lifestyle of *Feeling Fit*.

Linda Sorrells
Merry Anne Schmied

PROGRAM 1

Wellness: The Lifestyle of Feeling Fit

Wellness is a way of life, a lifestyle that *you* design in order to achieve your highest potential for well-being. Wellness is a *choice*. No matter what your present state of health, you can move to a higher level of wellness. Wellness involves self-acceptance and self-responsibility for living in a manner that serves you and doesn't undermine your health. Getting in touch with your own wellness lifestyle is the place to begin. The focus of each of the *Feeling Fit* videos is YOU.

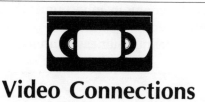

Video Connections

The film presented several characteristics of a wellness lifestyle. Answer the following questions related to your ideas of wellness.

1. Did the film present you with new wellness information you can use in evaluating your current lifestyle? Compare your thoughts on wellness with those presented by the wellness professionals in the film. _____

   _____

   _____

2. Are you doing all you can to be as healthy as possible? Are you willing to begin to learn more about wellness and to make modifications in your lifestyle? Can family, friends, and co-workers help you improve the quality of your life? _____

_____

_____

3. In the video Don Ardell made the point that the wellness lifestyle should have ''payoffs'' for the individual. List some payoffs you reap from your current lifestyle. Next, list payoffs you would like to achieve through the wellness way of life. _____

_____

_____

4. Al Shepston discussed a brief history of the wellness movement. State your own reasons why the wellness movement is gaining recognition by companies and individuals. ___

_____

_____

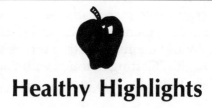

Healthy Highlights

- The treatment/medical model of health care attempts to return you to the state described in the neutral model.
- The wellness model tries to move you to a higher level of wellness.
- Approximately 48 percent of deaths are caused by unhealthy lifestyles, 24 percent by genetic defects and natural biology, 16 percent by environmental factors, and 12 percent by conditions that could have been treated.
- Where would you fall on the wellness-illness continuum? _____

_____

_____

You and Wellness: Self-Assessment

When you move toward a wellness way of life, you first must evaluate your current lifestyle. Begin by assessing how important each of the following dimensions is to you. How close does your present lifestyle come to meeting your needs in each dimension?

Dimension	Importance to me Great/Moderate/Little	Current lifestyle meets my needs Yes/No	If no, what strategies might I incorporate to improve?
INTELLECTUAL Stimulating mental activities			
EMOTIONAL Awareness and acceptance of my feelings			
PHYSICAL High level of vitality			
SOCIAL Contributions to my community			
OCCUPATIONAL Satisfaction from work			
SPIRITUAL Finding meaning in human existence			

Another method of assessing your lifestyle is to examine your behaviors on tests such as *Healthstyle*. This will help you evaluate your health knowledge and health habits.

HEALTHSTYLE A SELF-TEST

All of us want good health. But many of us do not know how to be as healthy as possible. Health experts now describe *lifestyle* as one of the most important factors affecting health. In fact, it is estimated that as many as seven of the ten leading causes of death could be reduced through common-sense changes in lifestyle. That's what this brief test, developed by the Public Health Service, is all about. Its purpose is simply to tell you how well you are doing to stay healthy. The behaviors covered in the test are recommended for most Americans. Some of them may not apply to persons with certain chronic diseases or handicaps, or to pregnant women. Such persons may require special instructions from their physicians.

Cigarette Smoking

If you *never smoke*, enter a score of 10 for this section and go to the next section on *Alcohol and Drugs*.

	Almost Always	Sometimes	Almost Never
1. I avoid smoking cigarettes.	2	1	0

	Almost Always	Sometimes	Almost Never
2. I smoke only low tar and nicotine cigarettes *or* I smoke a pipe or cigars.	2	2	3

Smoking Score: _____

Alcohol and Drugs

1. I avoid drinking alcoholic beverages *or* I drink no more than 1 or 2 drinks a day.   4 1 0

2. I avoid using alcohol or other drugs (especially illegal drugs) as a way of handling stressful situations or the problems in my life.   2 1 0

3. I am careful not to drink alcohol when taking certain medicines (for example, medicine for sleeping, pain, colds, and allergies), or when pregnant.   2 1 0

4. I read and follow the label directions when using prescribed and over-the-counter drugs.   2 1 0

Alcohol and Drugs Score: _____

Eating Habits

1. I eat a variety of foods each day, such as fruits and vegetables, whole grain breads and cereals, lean meats, dairy products, dry peas and beans, and nuts and seeds.   4 1 0

2. I limit the amount of fat, saturated fat, and cholesterol I eat (including fat on meats, eggs, butter, cream, shortenings, and organ meats such as liver).   2 1 0

3. I limit the amount of salt I eat by cooking with only small amounts, not adding salt at the table, and avoiding salty snacks.   2 1 0

4. I avoid eating too much sugar (especially frequent snacks of sticky candy or soft drinks).   2 1 0

Eating Habits Score: _____

Exercise/Fitness

1. I maintain a desired weight, avoiding overweight and underweight.   3 1 0

2. I do vigorous exercises for 15-30 minutes at least 3 times a week (examples include running, swimming, brisk walking).

3. I do exercises that enhance my muscle tone for 15-30 minutes at least 3 times a week (examples include yoga and calisthenics).   2 1 0

4. I use part of my leisure time participating in individual, family, or team activities that increase my level of fitness (such as gardening, bowling, golf, and baseball).   2 1 0

Exercise/Fitness Score: _____

Stress Control

1. I have a job or do other work that I enjoy.   2 1 0

2. I find it easy to relax and express my feelings freely.   2 1 0

3. I recognize early, and prepare for, events or situations likely to be stressful for me.   2 1 0

4. I have close friends, relatives, or others whom I can talk to about personal matters and call on for help when needed.   2 1 0

5. I participate in group activities (such as church and community organizations) or hobbies that I enjoy.   2 1 0

Stress Control Score: _____

Safety

1. I wear a seat belt while riding in a car.   2 1 0

2. I avoid driving while under the influence of alcohol and other drugs.   2 1 0

3. I obey traffic rules and the speed limit when driving.   2 1 0

4. I am careful when using potentially harmful products or substances (such as household cleaners, poisons, and electrical devices).   2 1 0

5. I avoid smoking in bed.   2 1 0

Safety Score: _____

What Your Scores Mean to You

Scores of 9 and 10

Excellent! Your answers show that you are aware of the importance of this area to your health. More important, you are putting your knowledge to work for you by practicing good health habits. As long as you continue to do so, this area should not pose a serious health risk. It's likely that you are setting an example for your family and friends to follow. Since you got a very high test score on this part of the test, you may want to consider other areas where your scores indicate room for improvement.

Scores of 6 to 8

Your health practices in this area are good, but there is room for improvement. Look again at the items you answered with a "Sometimes" or "Almost Never." What changes can you make to improve your score? Even a small change can often help you achieve better health.

Scores of 3 to 5

Your health risks are showing! Would you like more information about the risks you are facing and about why it is important for you to change these behaviors? Perhaps you need help in deciding how to successfully make the changes you desire. In either case, help is available.

Scores of 0 to 2

Obviously, you were concerned enough about your health to take the test, but your answers show that you may be taking serious and unnecessary risks with your health. Perhaps you are not aware of the risks and want to do something about them. You can easily get the information and help you need to improve, if you wish. The next step is up to you.

YOU Can Start Right Now!

In the test you just completed were numerous suggestions to help you reduce your risk of disease and premature death. Here are some of the most significant:

Score _____ **Avoid cigarettes**. Cigarette smoking is the single most important preventable cause of illness and early death. It is especially risky for pregnant women and their unborn babies. Persons who stop smoking reduce their risk of getting heart disease and cancer. So if you're a cigarette smoker, think twice about lighting that next cigarette. If you choose to continue smoking, try decreasing the number of cigarettes you smoke and switching to a low tar and nicotine brand.

Score _____ **Follow sensible drinking habits.** Alcohol produces changes in mood and behavior. Most people who drink are able to control their intake of alcohol and to avoid undesired, and often harmful, effects. Heavy, regular use of alcohol can lead to cirrhosis of the liver, a leading cause of death. Also, statistics clearly show that mixing drinking and driving is often the cause of fatal or crippling accidents. So if you drink, do it wisely and in moderation. *Use care in taking drugs*. Today's greater use of drugs—both legal and illegal— is one of our most serious health risks. Even some drugs prescribed by your doctor can be dangerous if taken when drinking alcohol or before driving. Excessive or continued use of tranquilizers (or "pep pills") can cause physical and mental problems. Using or experimenting with illicit drugs such as marijuana, heroin, cocaine, and PCP may lead to a number of damaging effects or even death.

Score _____ **Eat sensibly**. Overweight individuals are at greater risk for diabetes, gall bladder disease, and high blood pressure. So it makes good sense to maintain proper weight. But good eating habits also means holding down the amount of fat (especially saturated fat), cholesterol, sugar, and salt in your diet. If you must snack, try nibbling on fresh fruits and vegetables. You'll feel better— and look better, too.

Score _____ **Exercise regularly**. Almost everyone can benefit from exercise—and there's some form of exercise almost everyone can do. (If you have any doubt, check first with your doctor.) Usually, as little as 15-30 minutes of vigorous exercise three times a week will help you have a healthier heart, eliminate excess weight, tone up sagging muscles, and sleep better. Think how much difference all these improvements could make in the way you feel!

Score _____ **Learn to handle stress**. Stress is a normal part of living; everyone faces it to some degree. The causes of stress can be good or bad, desirable or undesirable (such as a promotion on the job or the loss of a spouse). Properly handled, stress need not be a problem. But unhealthy responses to stress—such as driving too fast or erratically, drinking too much, or prolonged anger or grief—can cause a variety of physical and mental problems. Even on a very busy day, find a few minutes to slow down and relax. Talking over a problem with someone you trust can often help you find a satisfactory solution. Learn to distinguish between things that are "worth fighting about" and things that are less important.

Score _____ **Be safety conscious**. Think "safety first" at home, at work, at school, at play, and on the highway. Buckle seat belts and obey traffic rules. Keep poisons and weapons out of the reach of children, and keep emergency numbers by your telephone. When the unexpected happens, you'll be prepared.

Where Do You Go From Here:

Start by asking yourself a few frank questions: *Am I really doing all I can to be as healthy as possible? What steps can I take to feel better? Am I willing to begin now?* If you scored low in one or more *sections* of the test, decide what changes you want to make for improvement. You might pick that aspect of your lifestyle where you feel you have the best chance for success and tackle that one first. Once you have improved your score there, go on to other areas.

If you already have tried to change your health habits (to stop smoking or exercise regularly, for example), don't be discouraged if you haven't yet succeeded. The difficulty you have encountered may be due to influences you've never really thought about—such as advertising—or to a lack of support and encouragement. Understanding these influences is an important step toward changing the way they affect you.

There's Help Available. In addition to personal actions you can take on your own, there are community programs and groups (such as the YMCA or the local chapter of the American Heart Association) that can assist you and your family to make the changes you want to make. If you want to know more about these groups or about health risks, contact your local health department or the National Health Information Clearinghouse. There's a lot you can do to stay healthy or to improve your health—and there are organizations that can help you. Start a new HEALTHSTYLE today!

For assistance in locating specific information on these and other health topics, write to the National Health Information Clearinghouse.

* National Health Information Clearinghouse
  P.O. Box 1133
  Washington, DC 20013

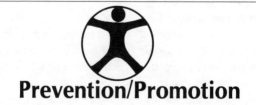

Prevention/Promotion

To a great extent, you determine the quality of your life. A person with no interest in taking steps toward greater wellness is a "preventer." A "promoter," on the other hand, takes the initiative in living a wellness lifestyle. Are you a preventer or a promoter of a high quality of life?

Preventer of High Quality of Life	Promoter of High Quality of Life

Identify six of your health habits and attitudes. Check (✓) whether they prevent or promote quality of life.

_____

_____

_____

_____

Family and friends can have both direct and indirect influences on the health habits you choose. List five family members or friends and indicate whether they are preventers or promoters.

_____

_____

_____

_____

When you strive to live a healthy lifestyle, support from significant people in your life is a must. Wellness can be a vehicle for families to spend more time doing things together. How can you create a more supportive environment?

_____

_____

_____

_____

What illnesses have you and your family had in the past year? Which might have been prevented by a wellness lifestyle?

_____

_____

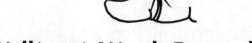

Well(ness) Worth Remembering

A wellness lifestyle includes the pursuit of activities that provide an increased number of positive payoffs; a wellness lifestyle is a richer way to live. The need for developing each dimension of wellness will vary considerably among people. For some, the happiness and satisfaction of high-level wellness come primarily from engaging in stimulating intellectual activities—for others, from the social or spiritual dimensions, which include a sense of purpose in reaching out to serve others. Remember the analogy of the three-legged stool offered by Susan Kern, assistant to the president of Illinois State University: The physical, mental, and emotional dimensions comprise the three legs of a stool; if you took away any one of the legs, the stool would fall over.

As you progress through the *Feeling Fit* series, continue to take close looks at your lifestyle. Identify areas that need to be modified and ways through which you can commit yourself to achieving HIGH-LEVEL WELLNESS.

PROGRAM 2

Lifestyle Risk Factors

Everyone wants to live life to the fullest. This dream, however, is dependent on many variables, such as health, finances, education, and opportunities. Now is the time to start developing a lifestyle that will insure that you can make the most of everything that comes your way. The more you know about how to improve the quality of your life, the better chance you have of making changes successfully.

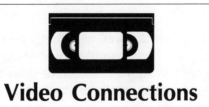

Video Connections

Social scientists and medical personnel looking at the leading causes of death have determined that approximately 50 percent of deaths are due to some type of heart disease.

1. The film stated that infectious disease is no longer the number one cause of death in the United States. What lifestyle changes in your generation have caused heart disease to be the number one killer? _____

_____

_____

2. Five risk factors for heart disease were discussed in the film. List them and place a check mark by any you have. _____

_____

_____

3. Is there any indication in your family history that you have the potential for developing any of the risk factors? _____

_____

_____

4. Develop a plan to avoid and modify these lifestyle risk factors. Compare your plan with the suggestions offered in the next video. _____

_____

_____

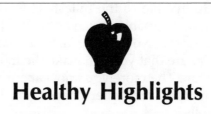

Healthy Highlights

- High Blood Pressure

  -tends to run in families;
  -tends to rise after puberty, especially in males;
  -is elevated by situations that are threatening or stressful.

- Cholesterol

  -is manufactured in your system as well as being absorbed from your diet;
  -can be lowered by twenty to thirty minutes of sustained exercise every other day;
  -is found in fats (animal fat has more cholesterol than plant fat does);
  -has been found deposited in artery walls in young teenagers, not only in older people, as was formerly thought;
  -buildup reflects poor dietary and exercise habits.

- Obesity

  -is a problem in about one fifth of the childhood population and increases with age;
  -causes added pressure on the circulatory system, because one pound of excess fat requires 200 miles of capillaries.

- Smoking

  -doubles the risk of a heart attack;
  -is a stimulant, raising the heart rate and constricting blood vessels;
  -has been linked to the buildup of fatty deposits in the arteries.

- Stress

  -is useful in moderation because it causes physiological reactions that aid performance;
  -symptoms need to be recognized so that stress-reducing tactics can be used.

Your Lifestyle Risk Factors: Self-Assessment

Men

Find the column for your age group. Everyone starts with a score of 10 points. Work down the page *adding* points to your score or *subtracting* points from your score.

		54 or Younger	55 or Older
		Starting Score **10**	Starting Score **10**

1. Weight

Locate your weight category in the table below. If you are in . . .

	54 or Younger	55 or Older
weight category A	Subtract 2	Subtract 2
weight category B	Subtract 1	Add 0
weight category C	Add 1	Add 1
weight category D	Add 2	Add 3
Equals		

2. Systolic Blood Pressure

Use the "first" or "higher" number from your most recent blood pressure measurement. If you do not know your blood pressure, estimate it by using the letter for your weight category. If your blood pressure is . . .

		54 or Younger	55 or Older
A	119 or less	Subtract 1	Subtract 5
B	between 120 and 139	Add 0	Subtract 2
C	between 140 and 159	Add 0	Add 1
D	160 or greater	Add 1	Add 4
	Equals		

3. Blood Cholesterol Level

Use the number from your most recent blood cholesterol test. If you do not know your blood cholesterol, estimate it by using the letter for your weight category. If your blood cholesterol is . . .

		54 or Younger	55 or Older
A	199 or less	Subtract 2	Subtract 1
B	between 200 and 224	Subtract 1	Subtract 1
C	between 225 and 249	Add 0	Add 0
D	250 or higher	Add 1	Add 0
	Equals		

4. Cigarette Smoking

If you . . .

(If you smoke a pipe, but not cigarettes, use the same score adjustment as those cigarette smokers who smoke less than a pack a day.)

do not smoke	Subtract 1	Subtract 2
smoke less than a pack a day	Add 0	Subtract 1
smoke a pack a day	Add 1	Add 0
smoke more than a pack a day	Add 2	Add 3

Final Score Equals ☐   **Final Score Equals** ☐

			Weight Category (lbs.)			
Your Height						
Ft	In		A	B	C	D
5	1	up to 123	124-148	149-173	174 plus
5	2	up to 126	127-152	153-178	179 plus
5	3	up to 129	130-156	157-182	183 plus
5	4	up to 132	133-160	161-186	187 plus
5	5	up to 135	136-163	164-190	191 plus
5	6	up to 139	140-168	169-196	197 plus
5	7	up to 144	145-174	175-203	204 plus
5	8	up to 148	149-179	180-209	210 plus
5	9	up to 152	153-184	185-214	215 plus
5	10	up to 157	158-190	191-221	222 plus
5	11	up to 161	162-194	195-227	228 plus
6	0	up to 165	166-199	200-232	233 plus
6	1	up to 170	171-205	206-239	240 plus
6	2	up to 175	176-211	212-246	247 plus
6	3	up to 180	181-217	218-253	254 plus
6	4	up to 185	186-223	224-260	261 plus
6	5	up to 190	191-229	230-267	268 plus
6	6	up to 195	196-235	236-274	275 plus
Estimate of Systolic Blood Pressure			119 or less	120 to 139	140 to 159	160 or more
Estimate of Blood Cholesterol			199 or less	200 to 224	225 to 249	250 or more

Weight Table for Men Look for your height (without shoes) in the far left column and then read across to find the category into which your weight (in indoor clothing) would fall.

Because both blood pressure and blood cholesterol are related to weight, an estimate of these risk factors for each weight category is printed at the bottom of the table.

Women

Find the column for your age group. Everyone starts with a score of 10 points. Work down the page *adding* points to your score or *subtracting* points from your score.

	54 or Younger	55 or Older
	Starting Score **10**	Starting Score **10**

1. *Weight*

Locate your weight category in the table below. If you are in . . .

	54 or Younger	55 or Older
weight category A	Subtract 2	Subtract 2
weight category B	Subtract 1	Subtract 1
weight category C	Add 1	Add 0
weight category D	Add 2	Add 1
Equals		

2. *Systolic Blood Pressure*

Use the "first" or "higher" number from your most recent blood pressure measurement. If you do not know your blood pressure, estimate it by using the letter for your weight category. If your blood pressure is . . .

		54 or Younger	55 or Older
A	119 or less	Subtract 2	Subtract 3
B	between 120 and 139	Subtract 1	Add 0
C	between 140 and 159	Add 0	Add 3
D	160 or greater	Add 1	Add 6
	Equals		

3. *Blood Cholesterol Level*

Use the number from your most recent blood cholesterol test. If you do not know your blood cholesterol, estimate it by using the letter for your weight category. If your blood cholesterol is . . .

		54 or Younger	55 or Older
A	199 or less	Subtract 1	Subtract 3
B	between 200 and 224	Add 0	Subtract 1
C	between 225 and 249	Add 0	Add 1
D	250 or higher	Add 1	Add 3
	Equals		

4. *Cigarette Smoking*

If you . . .

	54 or Younger	55 or Older
do not smoke	Subtract 1	Subtract 2
smoke less than a pack a day	Add 0	Subtract 1
smoke a pack a day	Add 1	Add 1
smoke more than a pack a day	Add 2	Add 4
Equals		

5. *Estrogen Use*

Birth control pills and hormone drugs contain estrogen. A few examples are: • Premarin • Ogan • Menstranol • Provera • Evex • Menest • Estinyl • Meurium

- Have your ever taken estrogen for five or more years in a row?
- Are you age 35 years or older and are now taking estrogen?

No to both questions	Add 0	Add 0
Yes to one or both questions	Add 1	Add 3

Final Score Equals ☐   Final Score Equals ☐

Your Height		Weight Category (lbs.)			
Ft	In	A	B	C	D
4	8	up to 101	102-122	123-143	144 plus
4	9	up to 103	104-125	126-146	147 plus
4	10	up to 106	107-128	129-150	151 plus
4	11	up to 109	110-132	133-154	155 plus
5	0	up to 112	113-136	137-158	159 plus
5	1	up to 115	116-139	140-162	163 plus
5	2	up to 119	120-144	145-168	169 plus
5	3	up to 122	123-148	149-172	173 plus
5	4	up to 127	128-154	155-179	180 plus
5	5	up to 131	132-158	159-185	186 plus
5	6	up to 135	136-163	164-190	191 plus
5	7	up to 139	140-168	169-196	197 plus
5	8	up to 143	144-173	174-202	203 plus
5	9	up to 147	148-178	179-207	208 plus
5	10	up to 151	152-182	183-213	214 plus
5	11	up to 155	156-187	188-218	219 plus
6	0	up to 159	160-191	192-224	225 plus
6	1	up to 163	164-196	197-229	230 plus
Estimate of Systolic Blood Pressure		119 or less	120 to 139	140 to 159	160 or more
Estimate of Blood Cholesterol		199 or less	200 to 224	225 to 249	250 or more

Weight Table for Women Look for your height (without shoes) in the far left column and then read across to find the category into which your weight (in indoor clothing) would fall.

Because both blood pressure and blood cholesterol are related to weight, an estimate of these risk factors for each weight category is printed at the bottom of the table.

What Your Score Means

0-4

You have one of the lowest risks of Heart Disease for your age and sex.

5-9

You have a low to moderate risk of Heart Disease for your age and sex but there is some room for improvement.

10-14

You have a moderate to high risk of Heart Disease for your age and sex, with considerable room for improvement on some factors.

15-19

You have a high risk of developing Heart Disease for your age and sex with a great deal of room for improvement on all factors.

20 & over

You have a very high risk of developing Heart Disease for your age and sex and should take immediate action on all risk factors.

Warning

- If you have diabetes, gout or a family history of heart disease, your actual risk will be greater than indicated by this appraisal.
- If you do not know your current blood pressure or blood cholesterol level, you should visit your physician or health center to have them measured. Then figure your score again for a more accurate determination of your risk.
- If you are overweight, have high blood pressure or high blood cholesterol, or smoke cigarettes, your long-term risk of heart disease is increased even if your risk in the next several years is low.

How to Reduce Your Risk

- Try to quit smoking permanently. There are many programs available.
- Have your blood pressure checked regularly, preferably every twelve months after age 40. If your blood pressure is high, see your physician. Remember blood pressure medicine is only effective if taken regularly.
- Consider your daily exercise (or lack of it). A half hour of brisk walking, swimming or other enjoyable activity should not be difficult to fit into your day.
- Give some serious thought to your diet. If you are overweight, or eat a lot of foods high in saturated fat or cholesterol (whole milk, cheese, eggs, butter, fatty foods, fried foods) then changes should be made in your diet. Look for the American Heart Association Cookbook at your local bookstore.
- Visit or write your local Heart Association for further information and copies of free pamphlets on many related subjects including:
  - Reducing your risk of heart attack.
  - Controlling high blood pressure.
  - Eating to keep your heart healthy.
  - How to stop smoking.
  - Exercising for good health.

Some Words of Caution

- If you have diabetes, gout, or a family history of heart disease, your real risk of developing heart disease will be greater than indicated by your RISKO score. If your score is high and you have one or more of these additional problems, you should give particular attention to reducing your risk.
- If you are a woman under 45 years or a man under 35 years of age, your RISKO score represents an upper limit on your real risk of developing heart disease. In this case your real risk is probably lower than indicated by your score.
- If you are a woman whose use of estrogen has contributed to a high RISKO score, you may want to consult your physician. Do not automatically discontinue your prescription.
- Using your weight category to estimate your systolic blood pressure or your blood cholesterol level makes your RISKO score less accurate.
  - Your score will tend to overestimate your risk if your actual values on these two important factors are average for someone of your height and weight.
  - Your score will underestimate your risk if your actual blood pressure or cholesterol level is above average for someone of your height or weight.

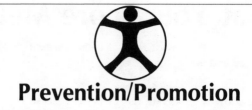

Prevention/Promotion

Do you make a sincere effort to reduce factors that put your heart at risk of disease? Circle the answers that best correspond to your case.

Preventer of Cardiovascular Health		Promoter of Cardiovascular Health
No	I restrict my intake of saturated fats.	Yes
No	I limit my intake of sodium.	Yes
No	I stay near my recommended weight.	Yes
No	I control my stress when it gets high.	Yes
No	I do not smoke.	Yes

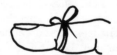

Well(ness) Worth Remembering

High blood pressure, high cholesterol levels, obesity, lack of exercise, stress, and smoking are all risk factors that can lead to heart disease. Exercise helps to lower blood pressure and blood cholesterol, aids in combating obesity, and is recommended for decreasing stress. Make exercise a part of your daily routine now so that it becomes a habit for life. Watch your diet and monitor your intake of animal fats. Be cholesterol-conscious. Develop a pressure valve for stress and learn when to use it; don't let stress be a risk factor for you.

Say no to smoking!

PROGRAM 3

Making Lifestyle Changes

Most people have habits that are keeping them from being as healthy as they could be. Although change is never easy, making lifestyle changes has major consequences in every aspect of life. The choices you make are based on how much you value certain areas of your life. You make choices continually: where to live, where to go to school, what clothes to wear, what friends to have, and what music to listen to. You also have choices about health: what to eat, what to drink, whether to smoke, how much to exercise, and how much to sleep. In today's program, you'll examine how certain lifestyle choices affect your commitment to feeling fit.

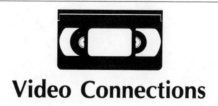

Video Connections

The film presented five steps necessary for successful lifestyle changes: assessment of current behavior, setting of goals, monitoring progress, rewarding yourself, and re-evaluating goals.

Assessment of Current Behavior

- Collect baseline information to help you understand your habits and determine your trouble spots (for instance, times of greatest stress or overeating).

- Many people feel they generally know what their problems are, but their descriptions may be too vague (e.g., overeating, tension).

Setting of Goals

- Set long-term goals that are realistic, specific, and measurable.
  SAMPLE LONG-TERM GOALS:
    Lose thirty pounds.
    Become more relaxed.
    Increase my activity.
- Set short-term goals that are realistic, specific, and measurable.
  EXAMPLES:
    Decrease daily consumption of soft drinks by 50 percent.
    Walk a mile at a brisk pace four days a week for the next month.

Monitoring Progress

- Keep a record of your behavior.
- Even though record-keeping is time-consuming, it increases the likelihood of success.

Rewarding Yourself

- Rewards are an important part of the behavior-changing process.
- Rewards can be internal (feeling self-esteem) or external (a certificate).
  SAMPLE REWARDS:
    Have someone else do the dishes.
    Call a friend for a long chat.
    Redo your hair.
    Listen to your favorite record.
    Wear a new jacket.
    Take pictures.
    Read a new book.
    Get a backrub.
    Buy new running shoes.
    Buy a wrench set.
    Buy a new dress.
    Go bowling.

Revising Your Goals

- If initial goals are too difficult, set easier goals or lengthen the time allowed to meet them.
- A continuing problem often is a sign that your goals are unrealistic.

1. Have you ever used any of these steps when trying to make changes? Were you successful? If not, why not? _____

   _____

   _____

2. Do you think the film has increased your chance of success in making desired changes?

   _____

   _____

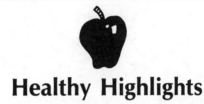

Healthy Highlights

Change Your Thinking

The American Lung Association has created what they call "self-talk." You can use "positive thinking" or self-talk to help cope with strong urges and develop the positive attitudes and self-perception that are important in successfully becoming a long-term nonsmoker, or making any other change.

Sample Situation:

   A co-worker asks me to join him, as usual, for a coffee break, which typically includes smoking.

NEGATIVE SELF-TALK:
- I'll never be able to resist and say no to a cigarette.
- I love sitting at the table with a cigarette and coffee at break.
- I don't want to hurt Al's feelings by not smoking with him.

POSITIVE SELF-TALK:
- I can resist smoking if I take one day at a time. It will get easier with time if I persist.
- I can relax better if I sit and chat over a cup of that new tea.
- I feel good when I stand up for what I believe in. This decision to quit is important to me.

You can apply self-talk to the lifestyle change you are trying to make. Recall some self-talk for the changes you are working on.

NEGATIVE SELF-TALK: _____

_____

POSITIVE SELF TALK: _____

_____

You and Lifestyle Change: Self-Assessment

Choose three behaviors you wish to change. Evaluate your ability and desire to change those specific behaviors.

Behavior:	Ability to Change				Desire to Change			
	low			high	low			high
_____	1	2	3	4	1	2	3	4
_____	1	2	3	4	1	2	3	4
_____	1	2	3	4	1	2	3	4

Select one behavior that you definitely are going to change.
   Example: Reduce soft drink intake to six ounces per day.

Collect baseline data during a three-day period.
   Example: Sunday, twenty-four ounces   Monday, eighteen ounces   Tuesday, twelve ounces.

Propose action.
   Example: Drink milk at lunch, limit the supply of soft drinks at home, drink more water.

Reinforce success.
   Example: Buy a new record if successful for five of the seven days.

Use helpful resources.
   Example: Talk with friends who discourage soft drink intake; keep juice in refrigerator at work.

Avoid barriers to success.
   Example: Be careful eating tacos and pizza, because soft drinks are enjoyable with those foods.

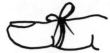

Well(ness) Worth Remembering

Identify the habits keeping you from being as healthy as you could be. Examine your lifestyle: Do you exercise regularly, eat well, avoid tobacco, manage stress effectively, and get enough sleep? Making lifestyle changes will help you live the most healthy, fulfilling life possible. Change requires information, along with love and support from people significant to you. It requires a carefully mapped-out plan and a chance to evaluate your success. It is important to set up appropriate short-term goals and rewards for achieving them. Most of what people do, both good and bad, is habitual, done without thinking—but you have choices. When you make a commitment to take care of yourself, you've made a major step toward better living. Consider a wellness way of life. Remember, your health is at the mercy of your lifestyle.

PROGRAM 4

Lifestyle Profiles

The process of making successful lifestyle changes requires careful planning and commitment. Making changes requires breaking old habits and developing new ones. In this program you heard the testimonies of three people who made healthy lifestyle changes that changed their lives. You do not have to wait until your problems are major; all you need is a desire to feel better and determination to reach your goals.

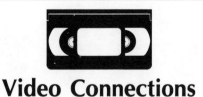

Video Connections

The film provided three true-life stories of people who overcame health problems by making lifestyle changes: Connie, who suffered from anorexia nervosa; Nora, who once weighed 243 pounds and slowly lost 94; and Cliff, who underwent triple-bypass surgery.

1. Do you know people who have similar problems? _____

_____

_____

2. Has the film helped you look at these problems in a different way? Explain. _____

_____

_____

3. Before you viewed the film, did you realize that eating disorders, overweight, and stress were such complex problems? _____

_____

_____

4. Now that you have heard a person tell about her experience with anorexia and bulimia, are you reminded of anyone who exhibits similar behaviors? If so, what could you do to help? _____

_____

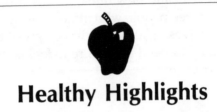

Healthy Highlights

Below are summaries of the three personal profiles you viewed. As you read them, circle the steps the person used in trying to make lifestyle changes. Remember, these steps involve assessment of current behavior, setting of goals, monitoring progress, rewarding oneself, and re-evaluating goals.

Profiles

Connie

Connie is a 5'4'', 22-year-old registered nurse who suffered from anorexia nervosa and bulimia for eight years. She had tried several on-again, off-again diets before becoming serious about losing weight. This meant near-starvation to Connie. She became totally obsessed with food, eating and then forcing herself to throw up.

Her goal was to get down to 100 pounds, first, then 90. She ultimately reached 80 pounds; However, she was not any happier. "I would look into the mirror, and all I saw was an enormous whale looking back at me. I hated myself. It was like a closet illness. I thought that I was the only person in the world who did this."

Connie would buy 20 dollars' worth of junk food, eat it, and then throw it up. She would ride along "restaurant row," stopping for food at every drive-up window. She would then feel so guilty she would force herself to throw up. Any feeling of stress could set off such an eating binge.

A newspaper advertisement for an eating disorders clinic brought Connie to the realization that she was not alone with this problem and that there was help available. She realized that her feelings of self-control were false and that the disorder was really controlling her, that she could hardly function because she was so obsessed with it.

A 6-week, in-patient clinic helped Connie make lifestyle changes and learn how to handle everyday stress. Connie has overcome her problem and now enjoys herself and life.

Nora

Nora is a 33-year-old project leader in computer programming and a mother of three. At 5'4'' and 243 pounds, Nora did not feel good about herself. She would eat anything, including a whole box of cookies at one sitting.

As a child, she was always overweight. At home she was required to clean her plate in order to get dessert; food was a reward. By the second grade she weighed 100 pounds. Nora had a very poor self-concept. ''As far as being a person, I wasn't a person . . . I just didn't exist that way.''

Then Nora decided to change her life. Her change was sparked by a friend who sent her a magazine on counting calories. Another friend encouraged her to start doing aerobics, which were part of an employee wellness program.

After losing 94 pounds, Nora credits exercise for keeping her weight down. Instead of avoiding exercise, she now seeks it every day. Also, she eats nutritiously; her diet includes lots of fruits and vegetables, but very little fried food or butter. Nora has planned a diet that works for both her family and herself; if necessary, she prepares herself a separate meal. At the start of her weight loss, Nora held strictly to a 1,000 calorie diet. She no longer counts calories, but *does* carefully watch what she eats. Foods such as chocolates are not sacrificed completely, but also are not overindulged in; furthermore, Nora no longer eats until her stomach feels full.

Nora stayed motivated by watching the numbers on the scale go down, being able to find clothes that fit, and finding low-calorie foods that tasted good. Nora is a new person, feeling much healthier and much better about herself.

Cliff

Cliff is a 53-year-old owner of a construction company who went through triple-bypass surgery. He had exercised regularly until 2 years before his heart attack. He experienced stress at work and ate an unhealthy diet.

Cliff's heart attack scared him greatly, and he was willing to do anything to get better. His limitations after surgery were difficult for him because he was used to having complete control over his company. Cliff chose bypass surgery over medication because it better assured him of the opportunity to return to the quality of life to which he was accustomed.

Cliff has made many lifestyle changes since surgery, including a 180-degree turnaround in his diet. Red meat and sweets have been nearly eliminated; he now eats a lot of fish, vegetables, and high carbohydrate foods. Cliff is now a firm believer in exercise, jogging 3 miles in the morning and feeling he can do things now that he had not done in 20 years—with energy to spare!

Cliff also has learned to lower his stress level. He no longer brings home his paperwork. He has learned to turn off his job until the next day.

Cliff feels fortunate he was able to change his lifestyle and enjoy his new life. He looks forward to the next 20 to 40 years.

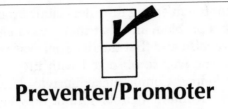

Preventer/Promoter

In program number three, you made plans for carrying out changes in three of your own behaviors. You can also be a very important part of someone else's efforts to make a lifestyle change. Think of someone you know who needs a lifestyle change. Write down four ways you can be a promoter and not a preventer of a healthy change.

Needed behavior change _____

What I can do to promote it: _____

_____

_____

_____

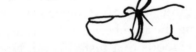

Well(ness) Worth Remembering

You can make any lifestyle change you want to. The task is not often an easy one; however, with a plan and a commitment to have a healthier body, you can accomplish your goals. You can also be a catalyst in helping others accomplish their goals. The result can be a life of feeling fit.

PROGRAM 5

You and Your Environment

The environment has a great influence upon your well-being. No matter what you do to promote your health, you will not be able to achieve a high level of wellness if you live in an unhealthy environment. When you think of an unsafe environment, you probably think first of air, water, and noise pollution. Although these can be very large-scale problems, you can do your part in helping to keep the environment a safe and healthy place to live in.

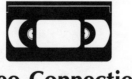

Video Connections

The film pointed out nine important characteristics of a healthy environment and related them to your well-being. Listed below are nine areas of environmental concern and what you as an individual can do about them.

Environmental Problem	Personal Control
Overpopulation	Limit the number of children in your family to two.
Air pollution	Follow recommended maintenance procedures for your car.
Proper disposal of wastes	Reduce or recycle household wastes. Buy multiple-use items instead of disposables. Do not litter. Support beverage container deposit legislation.
Toxic contamination	Limit use of pesticides around the home.
Food-borne disease	Understand proper food handling, nutrition, and ''time-temperature control'' principles.
Skin cancer caused by sun	Reduce your chance of skin cancer by covering exposed areas, using sunscreen, and not sunbathing between 11:00 a.m. and 2:00 p.m.
Indoor air pollution	Don't smoke, especially inside.
Noise pollution	Keep noise levels down and protect your hearing.
Environmental regulations	Become involved in the issues. Let elected officials know that you support regulations that promote the quality of life you want.

1. Had you considered how these areas of concern directly affect you? _____

_____

_____

2. Were you aware of how much refuse is generated by one person? _____

_____

_____

3. Do you know of someone who has been adversely affected by the environment, resulting in such problems as loss of hearing, food poisoning, or skin cancer? _____

_____

_____

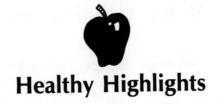

Healthy Highlights

Sixteen percent of all deaths follow illnesses caused or aggravated by environmental contaminants and stresses.

Damage to ears often is painless; thus people usually are not aware when they are hurting them. It is estimated that twenty million Americans are exposed to daily levels of noise which cause permanent damage.

Cigarette smoke is a major source of carbon monoxide, causing trouble ranging from headaches to death. By eliminating smoking, as much as 30 percent of the cancer deaths in the United States could be prevented.

Eighty percent of the illnesses in the world could be prevented if everyone had safe water.

Every pollutant going into the air remains in the "earth-atmosphere system" in some form. Vehicles are the main source of air pollution.

You and Your Environment: Personal Assessment

Define aspects of your environment that are not healthy and strategies that you can use to make them healthier.

Environmental Problem	How I Can Improve It
_____	_____
_____	_____
_____	_____

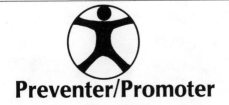

Preventer/Promoter

Are you a preventer or a promoter of a healthy environment? Circle the answers that best describe your behavior.

Preventer of a Healthy Environment		Promoter of a Healthy Environment
No	I properly dispose of litter.	Yes
No	I do not smoke.	Yes
No	Our household disposes of waste properly.	Yes
No	I keep my auto tuned properly.	Yes
No	I limit my exposure to loud music and noise.	Yes
No	I recycle materials when possible.	Yes
No	I make wise and limited use of pesticides.	Yes
No	I try to prevent overexposure to the sun.	Yes
No	I don't use aerosols.	Yes

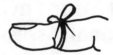

Well(ness) Worth Remembering

When you think in terms of the environment, you probably think of problems on a grand scale and out of your personal control. In fact, though, many of the risks you face are things over which you have considerable control. There is only so much air, water, and food to be used by the population of this planet. Everyone needs to be concerned about the proper use of these valuable resources. As the quality of resources deteriorates, so do people's health and well-being. This is already happening in Third World countries where water is unsanitary and there is not enough food. You must do your part in preserving a healthy environment.

PROGRAM 6

Stress and You

Stress is a part of daily life. It is a natural reaction of the body in response to pressure, real or imagined. Stress can have a positive rather than a negative effect if you understand how to control it.

If you want to manage stress successfully, you first must understand what it is and that your perceptions of stressors determine whether the result will be eustress (good stress) or distress (bad stress). You also must learn to recognize body signals that warn of overstress. A good understanding of stress leads to a healthier life.

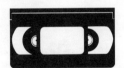

Video Connections

The video discussed stress and the "two Qs," the quality and quantity of life. Describe how stress has affected the quality and quantity of the lives of you and others you know.

1. The video pointed out that stressors can be used to your advantage. Can you think of a time when you let stress work for you, turning what could have been distress into eustress? _____

   _____

2. The video discussed Type A and Type B personalities. Review the characteristics of these personality types in relation to yourself. _____

   _____

   _____

Type A Characteristics	Type B Characteristics
• Extremely competitive with self and others	• Easygoing and patient
• Schedule- and time-oriented	• Worrying little about the future
• Moving and speaking quickly	• Making decisions based upon facts and common sense, not for the sake of professional status or social acceptance
• Goal-oriented, setting many goals at one time	• Setting realistic long-term goals, realizing that everything cannot be done at once
• Compulsively meticulous	• Not greatly critical of self and others
• Easily angered and upset	• Recognizing that petty irritations are part of life
• Hostile and aggressive	

3. Do you think your personality is predominantly Type A or Type B? Are there changes you wish to make in these characteristics? _____

_____

_____

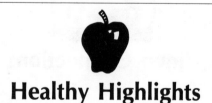

Healthy Highlights

A stressor is an occurrence that requires adaptation. Stress is a natural response of the body to a stressor. Your response to a stressor can be negative (distress) or positive (eustress). Eustress and distress cause the same physiological changes: Your heart beats faster, your blood pressure rises, and adrenaline and other hormones are secreted into the bloodstream.

Long ago, these changes were important as the ''fight or flight'' response; when an adversary approached, a person could either fight of flee the situation. Today this response is inappropriate in handling most stressors (such as your boss).

When you let several stressors cause distress, then you become overstressed. Distress can cause or contribute to such physical disorders as cancer, ulcers, colitis, heart disease, high blood pressure, migraine and tension headaches, and skin disorders. It can also cause such emotional reactions as crying, nervous tics, and worrying.

Stress and You: Self-Assessment

You often don't realize you are under stress. You need to listen to your body in learning to understand stress. Check the symptoms that you sometimes experience.

Stress Exhaustion Symptoms

Physical	Mental	Emotional
____ appetite change	____ forgetfulness	____ anxiety
____ headaches	____ low productivity	____ frustration
____ tension	____ negative attitude	____ the "blues"
____ fatigue	____ confusion	____ mood swings
____ insomnia	____ lethargy	____ bad temper
____ weight change	____ boredom	____ nightmares
____ digestive upsets	____ spacing out	____ crying spells
____ pounding heart	____ negative self-talk	____ irritability
____ proneness to accidents		____ feeling no one cares
____ teeth-grinding		____ depression
____ rashes		____ nervous laugh
____ restlessness		____ worrying
____ foot-tapping		____ discouragement
____ increased alcohol, drug, tobacco use		

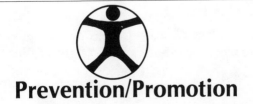

Prevention/Promotion

Do you promote, or prevent, good health by your understanding of stress? Answer the following questions to see where you lie on the health preventer-promoter continuum.

Preventer of Good Health		Promoter of Good Health
No	Do you know what causes stress for you?	Yes
No	Do you recognize your body's reactions to stress?	Yes
No	Do you have three or more characteristics of a Type B personality?	Yes

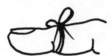

Well(ness) Worth Remembering

Stress is a part of everyday life. With too little stress you are bored; with too much stress, your body starts to wear down unless you learn to relax or handle the stress in a positive manner. By examining your perception of stressors and recognizing symptoms of stress and characteristics of a stressful personality, you can be in command of stress and let it work for you, not against you.

PROGRAM 7

Managing Your Stress

As many as 80 percent of illnesses are related to stress. You can improve your quality of life by recognizing your stressors and learning to cope with stress in a positive way.

   Once you recognize the stressors in your life, you must learn how to manage them so overstress does not wear down your body. You can prevent stress buildup by intervening in the stress cycle, which includes the stressor, your intrepretation of it, your body's physiological response, and your behavior in reaction to the stressor.

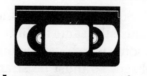

Video Connections

The video brought out how the same stressor can bring about different reactions in different people.

1. Can you think of a situation that you have perceived much differently from someone else?

   _____

   _____

2. The video also discussed how it is necessary to bring the body's responses down once stress starts adding up. Have you used such relaxation techniques as deep breathing, visualization, exercise, meditation, biofeedback, or muscular tension? If so, what was the situation and result? _____

   _____

   _____

The video introduced a three-step stress intervention strategy:

1. Change the situation.
2. Change your perception of the situation or of the stressor.
3. Change your reaction.

3. Which of these interventions do you use most often? Why do they work for you? ___
_____

_____

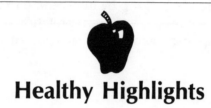

Healthy Highlights

Health professionals relate stress to 80 percent of all illnesses.

Although eustress and distress cause the same bodily changes, it is usually distress or hypostress (lack of stress, creating boredom) which causes illness.

Just as stress is very individualized, so must be strategies for coping.

Your perception of a stressor is one of the best stages at which to start managing stress. If you can interpret a stressor in a more positive way, it will not cause negative body responses.

Everyone experiences fifty to one hundred stressors per day, coping with 95 percent of them. The remaining 5 percent cause 95 percent of negative stress.

When stress occurs frequently or continuously and the physiological changes start to mount, you need a coping strategy to bring them back down. Without this relaxation, the body starts to wear down.

To cope with your stress, you must

1. recognize the stressors that you react to each day;
2. develop such coping strategies as:
   • changing the situation,
   • changing the way you think about the stressor or situation,
   • changing your physiological reaction.

Caffeine and nicotine bring on the same body changes as stress. Instead of promoting relaxation, they actually increase stress responses.

Managing Your Stress: Self-Assessment

List ten stressors that you have encountered in the past 24 hours. Indicate whether you experienced eustress or distress. Then indicate how you broke, or could have broken, the stress cycle. _____

	Type of Stress		Event or Situation		Perception or Interpretation			Physical Response				Behavior					
Stressor	Eustress	Distress	Leave Situation	Change Situation	Change Personality	Change Beliefs	Change Interpretation	Relaxation Techniques	Biofeedback	Exercise	Nutrition	New Coping Skills	Time Management	Communication Skills	Problem Solving Skills	Personal Management Skills	Assertion Training

Heading: **Coping Skills**

Person	Stressor	Coping Technique
_____	_____	_____
_____	_____	_____
_____	_____	_____
_____	_____	_____

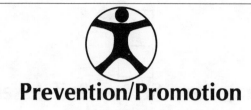

Prevention/Promotion

Remember, although it is virtually impossible to live without stress, you can be a promoter of eustress. Answer the following questions to see where you lie on the preventer-promoter continuum.

Preventer of Eustress		Promoter of Eustress
No	Can you find something positive in a stressful situation?	Yes
No	Can you relax when stress mounts?	Yes
No	Do you eat nutritiously and exercise?	Yes
No	Do you know what is really important to you and make your decisions accordingly?	Yes

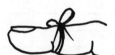

Well(ness) Worth Remembering

Only you can manage your stress. A stress management technique that works for one person may not work for another with the same type of stress. It is important for you to develop several different skills in managing stress because only certain strategies can be applied to a particular stressor. For example, if you are taking a test, you can't leave the situation, but you *can* use deep breathing techniques to relax. Stress management skills can add years to your life and life to your years.

PROGRAM 8

Exercise: A Way of Life

A complete physical fitness program must include activities that develop strength, flexibility, and cardiorespiratory endurance. With the advance of the high tech age, the average American lifestyle has become more sedentary. Americans' biggest killers, heart disease and cancer, are largely lifestyle related. Physical activity has become a popular trend in the past few years, with many people including regular activity programs in their lives. Exercise can reduce your risk of heart attack and stroke and can improve the quality of your life.

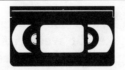

Video Connections

The video presented information on physical fitness and discussed psychological and physiological benefits of exercise.

1. List five physiological and five psychological benefits of exercise. _____

   _____

   _____

   _____

   _____

   _____

2. Has the video changed your mind about the importance of exercise for older people?

_____

_____

_____

3. Calculate your target heart rate according to the formula presented in the video.

4. While viewing the video, did you see any exercises that are not recommended? If so, which ones? _____

_____

_____

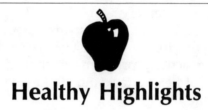

Healthy Highlights

Strength

- Strength is specific to each muscle group; therefore, each muscle group must be exercised to increase in strength.
- Strength decreases sharply with lack of use and gradually after age 35.
- An increase in overall strength takes 4-6 weeks to develop.
- Strength is increased by adding greater resistance, or more repetitions, or both, to a movement.

Flexibility

- Flexibility decreases if a joint is not used. It can be regained through use.
- Flexibility is increased by holding the musculature around a joint in a stretched position for 20-30 seconds.

Cardiorespiratory Endurance

- Endurance is gained by increasing the duration and/or the intensity of the specific activity.
- Endurance is developed by aerobic activity of 15 to 30 minutes duration, depending upon the physical condition of the individual.

Benefits of a Physical Activity Program

- Contributes to muscle strength, endurance, flexibility, and cardiorespiratory endurance.
- Helps to lower blood cholesterol.
- Helps to lower blood pressure.
- Contributes to weight control by burning additional calories.
- Aids in stress management by providing a change of pace for a person.
- Contributes to self-confidence as one sees and feels its results.
- Slows the loss of strength and flexibility that occurs with age.

Guidelines for an Activity Program

- The content should
  - -be a minimum of 20 to 30 minutes in length 3 to 4 times per week;
  - -include a warm-up of stretches, a main activity period, and a cool-down of stretches;
  - -be done in shoes that support the foot (weight-bearing activities);
  - -avoid the following exercises:
    - Toe touches with straight legs
    - Sit-ups with straight legs
    - Deep knee bends or full squats
    - Bouncing or jumping activities, if back or knee problems exist

How to Take Your Pulse

Taking your pulse accurately may require a little practice; however, learning to count your heartbeat correctly is critical in making an accurate assessment of your aerobic fitness.

- Place your fingertips on a carotid artery, which is on either side of the muscle running down the center of your neck. You can also measure your pulse on your radial artery, on the inside of your wrist on the thumb side (this pulse may be more difficult to find). Don't take your pulse with your thumb, because it has a pulse of its own, making it difficult to count the beats correctly.
- Press firmly but lightly; pressing too hard may actually slow your pulse rate.
- Count the beats for 10 seconds, then multiply by 6 to get the total number of beats for one minute. For example, if your heart beats 14 times in 10 seconds, your pulse is 84 beats per minute (6 times 14).
- Start counting your heartbeat at zero, not one. Count for 10 seconds. Have a helper take your pulse also. Compare the results; you may be pressing too hard or too lightly to get an accurate count.
- Cigarette smoking, caffeine intake, and stress affect your pulse rate.

You and Exercise: Self-Assessment

Rate your resting heart rate. The best time to do this is immediately upon waking, before rising from bed. Take your pulse for one minute by placing two fingers on your wrist or carotid artery. Record it and repeat every few weeks.

For an accurate pulse count at any time of the day, avoid drinking beverages containing caffeine or smoking for at least 2 hours beforehand. Your resting pulse is an indicator of your present level of aerobic fitness. How do you rate?

Very Fit	Fit	Average	Unfit
Under 55	56 to 69	70 to 84	85 and up

Rate the activity level in your lifestyle.

Sedentary	Low	Moderate	High

Determine your caloric needs based upon your activity level for a twenty-four-hour period.

Activity	Approximate Calories per Minute per Pound	Minutes	Pounds	Calories Needed
Sitting	.013	x	x	=
Walking	.018	x	x	=
Lying	.0078	x	x	=
Moderate exercising	.04	x	x	=

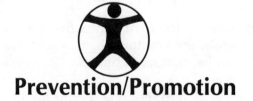

Prevention/Promotion

Activity is essential. The more sedentary your lifestyle, the higher your risk of developing heart disease. Which of these tactics will you use to increase your level of activity for the next week?

Prevent		Promote
No	Park several blocks from the office or store and walk the extra distance.	Yes
No	Take several walks during the workday, such as on breaks or at lunch.	Yes
No	Take stairs instead of elevators.	Yes
No	Walk or bike to the neighborhood store instead of taking the car.	Yes
No	Walk to the water fountain on a different floor instead of using the nearest one.	Yes

Your ideas:

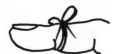

Well(ness) Worth Remembering

Remember, exercise is for the young at heart, and the only way to have a strong, young, healthy heart is to exercise. The more sedentary your lifestyle, the higher your risk of developing heart disease. Evaluate your present fitness level; by taking this first step, you are acknowledging the importance of physical fitness in achieving a rewarding life.

Maintaining an adequate fitness level will allow you the opportunity and satisfaction of experiencing full physical and mental power. No matter what your age, exercise will make you feel young, strong, and healthy. You will be less stressed and more able to enjoy a lifestyle of feeling fit.

PROGRAM 9

Individual Exercise Prescription

You are truly never too busy or too old to exercise. Daily activity is increasingly recognized as an essential element of a healthy life. People who have been physically inactive suddenly want to become active. Too often, though, they begin exercising and find the pace too fast or the activity unpleasant. Each person needs to determine where he or she stands in reference to age group standards, then to develop an individualized program of activity.

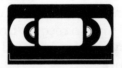

Video Connections

The film presented guidelines for establishing a good fitness program. It also discussed programs in China.

1. Did the film present information to help you evaluate your current program or those recommended through the media? _____

   _____

   _____

2. Did the film present any new ideas for fitness activities? Would you like to learn t'ai chi?

   _____

   _____

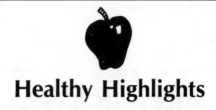

Healthy Highlights

Designing an Exercise Plan

- Select activities that are enjoyable, meet goal needs, and contribute to all of the components of physical fitness. A variety of activities can fulfill these requirements.
- Set aside a specific time for activity. There is no best time of day for everyone. In order for an exercise program to be successful it must be convenient.
- Plan for variety so that interest is maintained.
- If you can find someone else with similar activity needs, you should sometimes work together. This is a motivator.
- Be prepared to change activity levels as goals are met.

Guidelines for Your Program

- Determine your target heart rate. Formula: (220 − age) × 60 to 85 percent (percentage depends upon physical condition: low-level fitness, 60 to 65 percent; medium, 70 to 75 percent; high, 80 to 85 percent. Example: (220 − 20) × .70 = 140 beats per minute.
- Monitor your heart rate throughout the workout. Take your pulse for 10 seconds and multiply by 6 to get your heart rate per minute.
- Pay attention to your body signals. Pain or tenderness is a sign of stress to a joint or muscle. Stop to evaluate whether the intensity or frequency of the pain-causing activity is too great.
- Older individuals need additional time to recover from strenuous exertion. An every-other-day schedule best allows for recovery. A suggested pattern is a day of aerobic work alternating with a day of strength work.
- Start slowly. There is no magic in milestones or round numbers.
- Suggested time requirements for cardiovascular work:
    - *Warm-ups.* Five to ten minutes of stretches and gentle walking or slow jogging in order to prime the muscular and circulatory systems.
    - *Aerobic activity.* Fifteen to twenty minutes of jogging, swimming, fast walking, cycling, cross-country skiing, or aerobic dance.
    - *Cool down.* Five minutes of stretching, reducing muscle soreness, and allowing the body to return to its pre-exercise state.
- Suggested repetitions for strength development are six to eight per set at a given weight. When additional weight is added, the initial number of repetitions should be six.
- Suggested time limits for holding stretches (no bounces) is a minimum of 6 seconds and a maximum of 30 seconds.
- Include weight-bearing activities for arms.

- Wear well-fitted shoes with support, because many aerobic activities are weight-bearing for feet.
- Understand proper foot alignment. When jogging, land on the heel with feet pointed straight ahead. The weight transfer should be from the heel, along the outside border of the foot, to the ball of the foot.
- When possible avoid nonresilient surfaces, such as tile and concrete, which put extra stress on the ankle, knee, hip, and spine.

You and Your Individualized Exercise Plan: Self-Assessment

Find activities in which you participate on the following table and check out the fitness benefits.

Achieving Fitness Through Aerobic Exercise[1]

Program Type	Cardiovascular Fitness	Strength and Muscular Endurance	Flexibility	Body and Fat Control
Bicycling	***	**	*	***
Circuit overload training	**	***	*	**
Cooper's aerobics	***	*	*	***
Continuous calisthenics	***	**	***	***
Cross-country skiing	***	**	***	***
Dance aerobics	***	**	***	***
Hiking and backpacking	**	**	*	**
Jogging/running	***	*	*	***
Rope jumping	**	*	-	***
Swimming and water exercises	**	**	**	**
Walking	**	*	*	**

[1]Adapted from Anshel, Aerobics for Fitness

***Very good; **Good; *Minimum; -Low

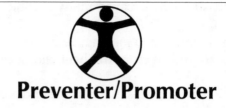

Preventer/Promoter

Are you feeling fit, or does your lifestyle prevent you from enjoying a life of fitness? Respond to the following statements to see if you are a preventer or a promoter of fitness.

Preventer of Fitness		Promoter of Fitness
No	I do vigorous exercises (running, brisk walking, biking, or swimming) for fifteen to thirty minutes at least three times a week.	Yes
No	I do exercises that enhance my muscle tone for fifteen to thirty minutes at least three times a week.	Yes
No	I know my target heart rate and try to stay within it when I exercise aerobically.	Yes
No	I use a warm-up and a cool-down as part of my exercise routine.	Yes
No	I use static stretching, rather than rebounding movements, to improve my flexibility.	Yes

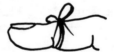

Well(ness) Worth Remembering

You had such good intentions; what are your excuses for not exercising? The film reviews four excuses and why they won't work anymore.

I Don't Have Time

This is the most used and abused excuse of all. Instead of singing this old tune, steal from other activities: take 3 minutes less in the tub, wake up 5 minutes earlier, take 3 minutes less reading the paper.

I Have to Watch the Kids

Exercise with the kids. If children grow up watching and joining in when their parents exercise, fitness becomes part of their lives.

I'm Too Tired

Nothing revs you up like proper exercise. Endorphins, which give you a feeling of euphoria, are released into the blood during exercise. Get high on exercise.

I'm Too Old

Today is the first day of the rest of your figure's life. At 45, you can't recontour your body to what it was at 18, but you can still make great improvements.

It's time to get moving and feeling fit.

PROGRAM 10

Nutrition and Your Lifestyle

Your quality of life depends to a great extent upon your nutritional choices, because you become what you eat. Many nutritional issues are clouded by conflicting emotions, scientific opinions, and consumer and producer interests. Should you reduce your intake of calories, fat, sugar, and cholesterol? Should you take a daily vitamin supplement? Are vegetarians more healthy than their meat-eating friends? What is the role of nutrients in the prevention of disease and extension of life? Some of this confusion exists because it is impossible to define a universal "ideal diet" meeting the needs of every individual.

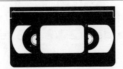

Video Connections

The film presented several dietary guidelines, as well as information on fast food, cholesterol, and sugar.

1. Did the film present new information to help you evaluate your diet? Compare your present food intake with these items: _____

_____

_____

2. Are you currently considering making any dietary changes? _____

_____

_____

3. How can you make eating at a fast food restaurant a more healthy experience? _____

_____

_____

4. The video discussed four benefits of eating a nutritionally sound diet in terms of controlling heart disease. How many benefits can you recall? _____

_____

_____

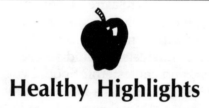

Healthy Highlights

Calcium

• Two out of three women over 17 do not get enough calcium.

Salt (Sodium)

• One's suggested daily sodium intake is 1,100 to 3,300 milligram (1/2 to 1 1/2 teaspoon). Many adults consume 6,000 milligram a day (2 1/2 to 3 teaspoon) which is too much.

Protein

• The average American eats more protein than necessary.

Sugar

• A sweet treat may pick you up, but it may also make your blood sugar plunge. Sweets initially raise the level of sugar in the blood, causing the body to produce extra insulin. Insulin rapidly removes sugar from the bloodstream, which may leave you worse off in terms of energy, mood, and hunger than you were before your treat.

Recommended Daily Dietary Allowances (RDA's)

| Persons | | | | | Minerals | | | | | | | |
Sex	Age Years From–To	Weight Pounds	Height Inches	Food Energy Calories	Calcium Milligrams	Phosphorus Milligrams	Iron Milligrams	Vitamin A International units[1]	Thiamin Milligrams	Riboflavin Milligrams	Niacin Milligrams	Ascorbic Acid Milligrams
Males	15 18	134	69	3,000	1,200	1,200	18	5,000	1.5	1.8	20	45
	19 22	147	69	3,000	800	800	10	5,000	1.5	1.8	20	45
	23 50	154	69	2,700	800	800	10	5,000	1.4	1.6	18	45
	51+	154	69	2,400	800	800	10	5,000	1.2	1.5	16	45
Females	15 18	119	65	2,100	1,200	1,200	18	4,000	1.1	1.4	14	45
	19 22	128	65	2,100	800	800	18	4,000	1.1	1.4	14	45
	23 50	128	65	2,000	800	800	18	4,000	1.0	1.2	13	45
	51+	128	65	1,800	800	800	10	4,000	1.0	1.2	12	45

Adapted from "Nutritive Value of Foods," United States Department of Agriculture, *Home & Garden Bulletin #72.*

[1]5 International Units = 1 Retinol Equivalent.

You and Nutrition: Self-Assessment

Record your food intake during a twenty-four hour period. You need to keep accurate track of the exact amount of each serving.

Food	Portion Size	Protein	Fat	Carbohydrate	Iron	Calcium	Calories	Changes Needed*
Breakfast								
Snack								
Lunch								
Snack								
Dinner								
Snack								
Total								

*Changes needed: (1) substitute foods, (2) modify foods, (3) eat smaller portions, (4) eliminate high-calorie foods.

As you review your 24-hour dietary record, check to see whether you were getting foods from all four basic food groups.

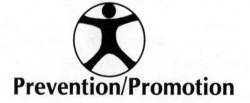

Prevention/Promotion

Research has indicated that many life-threatening diseases are strongly linked to food. Take this quiz to see if your diet prevents or promotes wellness:

Preventer of Wellness		Promoter of Wellness
Three or less	How many days each week do you eat two or more servings of fruits and two or more servings of vegetables?	Four or more
Three or less	How many days each week do you eat at least one fruit or vegetable high in vitamin C?	Four or more
Three or less	How many days each week do you eat at least one fruit or vegetable high in vitamin A?	Four or more
Three or less	How many days each week do you eat four servings of grain products?	Four or more
Three or less	How many days each week do you eat two or more servings of dairy products?	Four or more
No	Do you usually trim visible fat from meat before and after cooking?	Yes
No	Do you usually use soft (tub) margarine instead of butter or stick margarine?	Yes
Four or more	How many servings of baked goods do you eat each week?	Three or less
Five or more	How many times per week do you consume candy, soft drinks, or ice cream?	Four or less
Four or more	How many alcoholic drinks do you consume each week, on the average?	Three or less

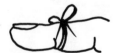

Well(ness) Worth Remembering

The importance of making educated consumer choices when selecting foods is an important aspect of proper nutrition and good health. When selecting food for yourself and your families, you should read package labels for the amount of fat, sodium, and calories per serving. Good nutrition is centered on good eating habits based on moderation and variety. You should use these seven guidelines to reach your goals:

- Eat a variety of foods.
- Maintain your ideal body weight.
- Avoid too much fat, saturated fat, and cholesterol.

- Eat foods with adequate starch and fiber.
- Limit sugar intake.
- Limit your sodium consumption.
- If you drink alcohol, do so in moderation.

By following these guidelines, you will reduce your risk of developing heart disease; you will be eating a diet for feeling fit.

PROGRAM 11

Weight Control

The key to weight control is lifestyle control. Maintaining your ideal weight and appropriate percentage of body fat involves good nutrition, exercise, and behavior modification.

Are Americans obsessed with losing weight? It seems so, considering the variety of books, magazines, exercise videos, and advertisements for pills, gadgets, and diet plans to help one lose weight, and lose it fast. You've read, ''Now you can burn away your ugly unwanted cellulite in 10 days.'' There are even claims of losing 10 pounds in less than a week. Getting to the truth concerning weight control is difficult.

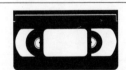

Video Connections

The film presented several theories of the cause of obesity. Here are three common ones.

Setpoint Theory

- The brain chooses the amount of body fat it considers ideal for your needs.
- The brain works to maintain that level of fat, the ''setpoint,'' by
  -increasing or decreasing your appetite,
  -prompting the body to waste excess energy if you overeat and conserve energy if you eat too little.

Brown Fat Theory

- The cause of obesity is the inability of an individual's brown fat to burn calories.
- Brown fat of overweight people may be inefficient or too limited in quantity to aid in maintaining normal weight.

Fat Cell Theory

- The cause of obesity is an excess number of fat cells.
- The number of fat cells is inherited, but can be increased by childhood overeating.

1. How do these theories compare to those you currently hold? _____

_____

_____

2. Some of the factors that contribute to obesity are controllable and others aren't. List two uncontrollable factors and at least five controllable ones. _____

_____

_____

3. Did the film present you with new information with which to evaluate weight loss quackery? _____

_____

_____

4. Did the film present any facts that changed your thoughts about your body weight and percentage of body fat? _____

_____

_____

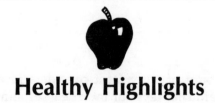

Healthy Highlights

One out of five persons is obese. These scales represent the minimum degree of obesity:

Male Obesity Scale		Female Obesity Scale	
Height	*Weight* (pounds)	*Height*	*Weight* (pounds)
5'6''	174	5'2''	150
5'8''	181	5'4''	157
5'10''	188	5'6''	164
6'	196	5'8''	172
6'2''	205	5'10''	179

- Aerobic exercise reduces fat in the abdominal area more than sit-ups.
- An inadequate intake of food can trigger the body's starvation defenses.
- Activity increases lean body tissue percentage and the body's ability to use calories.

Recognizing Quackery

It is easy to recognize quackery just by keeping your eyes open. Each ad uses one or more of the following types of claims:

- quick and easy cures
- natural ingredients
- scientific breakthroughs
- glowing testimonials

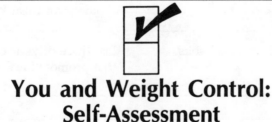

You and Weight Control: Self-Assessment

In the video you watched, Fred was weighed underwater to determine his percentage of body fat. Because hydrostatic weighing requires special equipment, other ways of estimating body fat have been developed.

1. The greater the ratio of your waist measurement to your hip measurement, the greater the risk for heart disease. Calculate your own ratio as shown in the following example:

$$\frac{\text{(waist measurement)} = 30''}{\text{(hip measurement)} \;\;= 40''} = .75$$

Use the following values to compare your score:

1.0 highest level for healthy men
.8 highest level for healthy women

2. Determine the ideal weight and percentage of body fat for your frame size by having your skinfold measurements taken.
3. Determine your daily caloric needs with the following guidelines:

(Female) Present weight _____ × 12 = _____

(Male)   Present weight _____ × 15 = _____

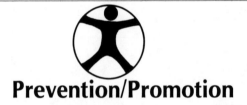

Prevention/Promotion

Prevent, so you won't have to repent! Your lifestyle can either promote ideal weight or prevent it.

Preventer of Ideal Weight	Promoter of Ideal Weight
List three of your eating and exercise habits that prevent ideal weight.	List three of your eating and exercise habits that promote ideal weight.
_____	_____
_____	_____
_____	_____

What changes would help you reach your ideal weight?

Physical Activity   Eating Habits

_____   _____

_____   _____

_____   _____

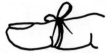

Well(ness) Worth Remembering

One out of five Americans is obese. Twenty million Americans are on a diet—and twenty million more think they should be. Of people losing weight, 80 percent will regain what they lost.

Getting to the truth concerning weight control is difficult, particularly with the bombardment of so many claims and gimmicks in this "body beautiful" world. This program has separated fact from fiction and reality from fantasy to find the truth about weight control. Maintaining a good body weight requires a lifetime commitment from you.

PROGRAM 12

Your Individual Diet Plan

Most people need to change their eating habits to decrease sugar, salt, and fat and increase fiber, iron, and calcium. Most people know which foods are good for health and which aren't, that too much fat, sodium, sugar, and caffeine is bad, and that fruit, vegetables, and whole grains are good. Three things often get in the way of intentions to eat right: busy lifestyles, obsession with thinness, and a lack of knowledge about the ingredients in processed foods.

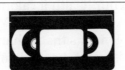

Video Connections

The film presented information about the psychological aspects of eating, obesity, overweight, and body composition.

1. Was food used to show love and provide rewards in your family? _____
_____
_____

2. Did the film present you with new information on the difference between obesity and overweight? _____
_____
_____

3. Are you obese, overweight, underweight, or ideal? _____

   _____

   _____

4. The members of the weight loss class at Carle Clinic all had stories to tell about their eating habits before dieting using behavior modification. Define behavior modification. Have you ever used this technique when dieting? _____

   _____

   _____

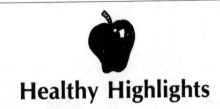

Healthy Highlights

- Weight loss through dieting alone results in loss of fat and muscle. Weight loss through activity consists almost entirely of body fat loss.
- Muscle tissue weighs more than fat. You can be losing fat and inches on a good diet and exercise program, but you might not be able to tell from your scale.
- Government guidelines recommend that 15 percent of calories come from protein, 30 percent from fat, and 55 percent from carbohydrates.
- Some nutrients in which many Americans are deficient are calcium, iron, and vitamins A, B, and C.
- Taking vitamins will not protect your health if caloric intake is severely restricted. Without food to metabolize, vitamins are usually wasted. You must eat well to stay healthy.
- There are no magic foods or supplements that enhance athletic performance. Much money is wasted on kelp, garlic, brewer's yeast, bee pollen, bone meal, lecithin, dessicated liver, and ginseng.

You and Your Diet: Self-Assessment

Re-evaluate your 24-hour food intake, as recorded in Program 10. Compare the percentages of calories comprised of carbohydrates, protein, and fat with the recommended amounts.

Calories/Nutrients	Recommended	Actual
Calories		
% Fat		
% Protein		
% Carbohydrates		
Iron		
Calcium		

Plan an individual diet based upon your suggested daily calorie intake (use the food exchange guide below.)

Breakfast _____

_____

Lunch _____

_____

Dinner _____

_____

Snacks _____

_____

Daily Caloric Food Plan Guide

Food	Number of Exchanges per Daily Food Plan					
	1,200 Calories	1,500 Calories	1,800 Calories	2,100 Calories	2,300 Calories	2,500 Calories
Vegetables	1	1	2	2	2	2
Breads	4	5	6	7 1/2	10	10
Meats	5	6	7	8	8	9
Milk	2	2	2 1/2	2 1/2	2 1/2	3
Fruits	4	4	4	6	6	6
Fats	1	4	5	6	7	8

If you desire a diet for 3,000 calories, double the diet suggested in the 1,500 calories list.

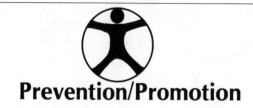

Prevention/Promotion

You can probably identify something in your diet that needs to be changed, but it is also important to realize that many of your current food choices are good ones. Eating well probably doesn't require a drastic overhaul of your habits.

   List your three favorite foods. Using a food content chart, rate each on its content of salt, sugar, fat, and fiber. Are you a preventer or promoter of nutritional health?

Preventer of Nutritional Health		Promoter of Nutritional Health
	Food	
Salt high		Salt low
Sugar high		Sugar low
Fat high		Fat low
Fiber low		Fiber high
Salt high	Salt low	Salt low
Sugar high		Sugar low
Fat high		Fat low
Fiber low		Fiber high
Salt high		Salt low
Sugar high		Sugar low
Fat high		Fat low
Fiber low		Fiber high

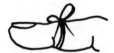

Well(ness) Worth Remembering

Authorities advise how to eat to win athletic events and urge changing eating habits to lower the risk of heart attack and cancer. Two simple principles are common to most of these dietary recommendations: reduce fat and increase fiber.

The experts say one thing over and over again. Whether your goal is to lose weight, improve your diet, or increase your exercise, to be successful you have to change your behavior. Changing any behavior that has become a habit works best when you follow these steps:

1. assess your behavior,
2. set a goal,
3. monitor your progress,
4. reward yourself for progress, and
5. revise your goals.

The most successful diet allows you to make a lifestyle change that you can live with—a food plan that you can stay on for years.

PROGRAM 13

Aging and Your Lifestyle

The quality of your life during old age depends to a great extent upon the lifestyle decisions that you make when younger. Aging is a gradual and natural process that begins at birth. By increasing your awareness of the changes that occur with aging, you can better influence the health status of your later years.

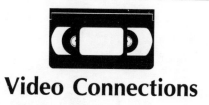

Video Connections

This film presents three aspects of aging: physical, mental, and social.

1. Describe some of the physical, mental, and social components of aging. Can leading a healthy lifestyle do anything to alter these processes? _____

   _____

   _____

2. Describe some of the myths about aging. Do you believe any of them? Did the film present you with new information to help you in evaluating these myths? _____

   _____

   _____

3. Did you know that an active 70-year-old has the same functional capacity as an inactive 30-year-old? _____

_____

_____

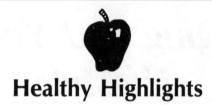

Healthy Highlights

- Twenty to 40 percent of aging is determined by genetic (primary) factors.
- Sixty to 80 percent of aging is determined by environmental factors such as lifestyle (secondary).
- Genetic and environmental factors can be slowed—and some secondary factors prevented—if you practice good nutrition, exercise regularly, control your weight, manage stress, and avoid smoking.
- Exercise is important at all ages, but it is *essential* in the later years.
- An active 70-year-old has the same functional capacity as a sedentary 30-year-old.
- Two-thirds of American women over age 17 do not receive enough calcium in their diets. Remember, insufficient amounts of calcium and exercise are primary causes of osteoporosis. osteoporosis.
- We age psychologically and sociologically, as well as physically. By developing a positive perspective of the aged and your own aging, you will enjoy a healthier old age.

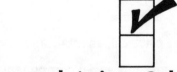

You and Aging: Self-Assessment

List four words or phrases that you associate with aging and the elderly.

_____

_____

_____

_____

Examine these words. Do they reflect a positive or negative attitude? (If in a group, share your thoughts.)

_____

_____

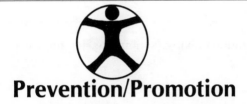

Prevention/Promotion

The following survey will help you determine if you and a member of your family are promoting or preventing healthy aging for yourselves. Circle the most accurate responses to the statements.

Preventer of Healthy Aging			Promoter of Healthy Aging	
You	*Family Member*		You	*Family Member*
No	No	I perform aerobic exercise* at least 3 times per week for 20 minutes or more.	Yes	Yes
No	No	I take at least 5 minutes per day to stretch my body.	Yes	Yes
No	No	I do not smoke.	Yes	Yes
No	No	I drink no more than an average of one alcoholic beverage per day.	Yes	Yes
No	No	I can control my stress level and bring it down if it gets high.	Yes	Yes
No	No	There is no history of cancer, stroke, heart attack, osteoporosis, arteriosclerosis, or arthritis in my family.	Yes	Yes
No	No	My calcium intake level** is adequate (premenstrual women, 1,000 to 1,200 milligram; postmenstrual women and elderly men, 1,500 milligram; all others, 800 milligram).	Yes	Yes
No	No	My caffeine intake*** is low (less than 200 milligram).	Yes	Yes
No	No	My cholesterol level is low (age 40 and under, less than than 200 milligram; older, less than 250 milligram).	Yes	Yes
No	No	I am not overfat. (If percentage of body fat is unknown, read, "I am not overweight."	Yes	Yes
No	No	I eat the recommended daily servings from the four food groups.****	Yes	Yes

Identify habits in your lifestyle that either prevent or promote healthy aging. List two changes you can make in your lifestyle in order to promote healthy aging. ___

_____

_____

How can you implement changes in the behaviors that you have identified and would like to change? _____

_____

_____

*Aerobic exercise includes strenuous biking, swimming, jogging, walking, and dance.

**Calcium content in foods:

1 cup milk	300 milligram	1 piece cake, pie, muffin	50 milligram
1 cup other milk product	200	2 eggs	50
1 ounce cheese	200	3/4 cup legumes cooked	50
1 cup dark leafy greens, broccoli, bok choy	200	1 ounce milk chocolate candy	50
1 cup cream soup	175		

***Caffeine content in foods:

12 ounce average soft drink (unless decaffeinated, such as 7-up, Pepsi Free, Sprite)	45 milligram	Instant iced tea	75 milligram
		Instant hot tea	30
		Brewed black tea	
Chocolate bar	25	weak	30
Brewed coffee	85	medium	60
Instant coffee	60	strong	90
		Cocoa	50

****Recommended servings of food groups:

Food Group	Teens	Adults
Dairy products	4	2
Meat and protein	2	2
Fruits and vegetables	4	4
Grains	4	4

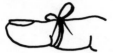

Well(ness) Worth Remembering

Aging doesn't begin at 30, 40, 65, or any other birthday; it begins at birth. You can greatly influence today how healthy you will be in your later years. It is never too late to start. Look to your future by promoting healthy lifestyle habits now.

PROGRAM 14

Longevity: How Long Will You Live?

Lifestyle is the most significant determinant of longevity. By eating better, exercising regularly, and eliminating smoking, you can live a longer and more productive life.

This program looks at the factors that influence your life expectancy. It emphasizes the importance of developing healthy lifestyle habits early in life, so that your later years will be healthy, happy, and productive.

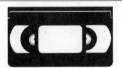

Video Connections

1. The video brought out several factors that influence how long you live. List some factors that will lead to a healthy, happy old age. _____

   _____

   _____

2. Taking these factors into consideration, how long do you think you might live, and why? Look through several newspapers to find the causes of deaths. Were they lifestyle related or uncontrollable? _____

   _____

   _____

3. Some common fears of the elderly were discussed in the video. List at least five of them.

_____

_____

4. The film mentioned the adjustment to retirement that must be made. Have you given much thought to how life will be once you retire? _____

_____

_____

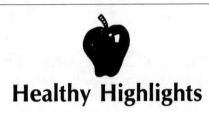

Healthy Highlights

- More people are living longer than ever before. The average life expectancy in the U.S. is 74.2 years (males, 70.8; females, 78.2).
- The human lifespan (biological limit to life) is 110 to 120 years.
- The majority of early deaths are caused by accidents or lifestyle-related diseases.
- Psychosocial, environmental, and lifestyle factors are more important determinants of health and longevity than are genetic and natural biological factors.
- The most important contributing factors to early death are
    - being obese or overweight,
    - poor nutritional habits,
    - excessive stress,
    - living a sedentary lifestyle,
    - smoking.
- Follow these seven basic health guidelines, which can add years to your life:
    - Eat regularly scheduled meals each day—no snacking.
    - Eat breakfast every day.
    - If you drink alcoholic beverages, do so in moderation.
    - Exercise regularly.
    - Moderate your weight.
    - Sleep seven to eight hours each night.
    - Do not smoke.
- It's never too late to start good nutrition and physical exercise.
- Proper dietary practices may increase your life by five to ten years.
- Proper exercise helps you maintain your ideal body weight and an efficient and healthy cardiovascular system.

- Exercise also helps maintain your mobility, thus enabling you to be socially active in later years. A good social support system enhances health and longevity.
- Exercise helps improve older persons' self-esteem.
- Stress is the primary determinant of whether an average life expectancy is attained. The elderly encounter stressors such as loneliness, retirement, financial hardship, and pain. The better prepared they are to deal with these stressors, the less likely it is that they will succumb to early illness and death.
- Having good relationships, reaching out and not expecting other people to take all of the initiative, will increase the possibility of a healthy, happy, productive, and long life.

How Long Will You Live?: Self-Assessment

Record your family history by filling in the blanks as completely as possible.

Family History of _____
(your name)

Name	Current Age or Age at Death	Year of Death	Cause of Death
Brother/sister			
Brother/sister			
Brother/sister			
Mother			
Father			
Maternal Grandmother			
Maternal Grandfather			
Paternal Grandmother			
Paternal Grandfather			
Great Grandparent			
Great Grandparent			

Using your family history, determine the average age of death of your relatives _____ _____; whether the types of causes of death have changed over the years. Explain _____

_____

What illnesses run in your family that you can help prevent by lifestyle decisions? What changes do you need to make? _____

_____

_____

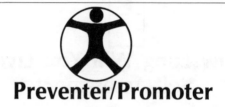

Preventer/Promoter

Are you doing all you can to promote a longer and healthier life? Circle the answers that pertain to you.

Preventer of Longevity		Promoter of Longevity
	Genetic Factor (Uncontrollable)	
No	My ancestors were long-lived.	Yes
	Lifestyle and Psychosocial Factors (Controllable)	
No	I eat three healthy meals and no snacks.	Yes
No	I do not smoke.	Yes
No	I get seven to eight hours of sleep a night.	Yes
No	I exercise regularly three or more times a week.	Yes
No	I have a good social support system.	Yes
No	I maintain a useful and satisfying role in society.	Yes

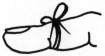

Well(ness) Worth Remembering

The decisions you make about the lifestyle you lead will to a great extent determine your well-being in your later years. They will also have a bearing upon how long you will live.

Remember, the three most important ways to increase your life expectancy are by

- maintaining a useful and satisfying role in society,
- maintaining good physical functioning,
- avoiding smoking.

PROGRAM 15

New Horizons

Each person can make individual choices that lead to optimal wellness. To make the decisions, you need to be aware of new technologies and environmental and societal forces that will influence your choices.

Think of a world free of illness, a world with doctors and hospitals whose objective is to help disease-free persons reach optimal levels of health and fitness. Consider a world where scientists can change the heredity of human beings by removing or adding genes to fertilized eggs, thus creating "humans by design." These changes are on the horizon.

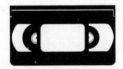

Video Connections

The film presented information about the future direction of health promotion and the wellness lifestyle.

1. What does the future hold for the wellness movement? _____
   _____
   _____

2. What needs to be done so that every American can enjoy a wellness lifestyle? _____
   _____
   _____

3. What do you think are the most promising areas of research for improving the quality and length of life? _____

_____

_____

4. What are the moral implications of genetic engineering? _____

_____

_____

5. What do you feel are governmental and private organizations' roles in health promotion?

_____

_____

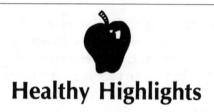

Healthy Highlights

Genetic Engineering

- There are approximately 100,000 genes inside each human cell.
- Scientists have isolated 21,500 of these genes and have identified their specific functions, such as regulating the production of insulin or causing cancer.
- In 10 to 20 years, scientists probably will have identified all human genes and will be able to cure many diseases by altering genes (gene replacement therapy).
- Scientists already use biotechnology to produce many enzymes and hormones, such as insulin, growth hormones, and neurotransmitters.
- Synthetic and recombinant DNA vaccines will fight hepatitis B, herpes, gonorrhea, chicken pox, malaria, typhoid, diphtheria, cancer, and rabies virus.

Other Likely Medical Advances

- It will be possible to replace such body parts as blood vessels, nerve cells, brain cells, and hormone-producing cells. This will prevent the need for amputations and will provide cures for Alzheimer's disease and other illnesses.
- It will be possible to regenerate injured nerve cells in the brain and spinal cord.
- Immune system stimulants will enhance cancer treatments and prevent or reverse such degenerative muscular disorders as multiple sclerosis and muscular dystrophy.

- New drugs will be more predictable and specific in their actions. Monoclonal antibodies attack specific viruses, and nothing else, whereas old antibodies attack many substances. Even the common cold may be defeated by certain monoclonal antibodies.
- Doctors can already replace the heart, ear, blood vessels, limbs, pancreas, kidneys, and joints. Many more body parts will be replaced by plastic and bionic parts.

Predictions for a Baby Born in 1986

He or she

- will be more likely to live to 100 years of age (life expectancy will be about 75 for men and 83 for women);
- will be largely free of physical and mental disease;
- will be vaccinated against everything from tooth decay to herpes;
- will enjoy a greatly improved quality of life;
- will be concerned with dangerous environmental pollutants;
- will retire at a later age;
- will see the common use of such reproductive interventions as *in vitro* fertilization or embryo transfer;
- will have more time for leisure, as a result of a shorter work week.

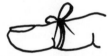

Well(ness) Worth Remembering

With proper health promotion education, today's youths will have the tools and motivation to lead long, productive, and healthy lives. Yet, no matter what your age or present lifestyle, you should consider a wellness lifestyle for three basic reasons.

First, illness can be dangerous and extraordinarily expensive disruptions of your life. Fortunately, you can avoid most of them (the second reason). Aging is negotiable to the extent that you take good care of yourself. The third reason is perhaps the most persuasive: living in a manner consistent with your own unique approach to wellness is a richer way to be alive and is its own reward.

The wellness movement offers proven principles and concepts for living a better life; yet, much work needs to be done for the wellness movement to become completely successful. Government, business, the medical professions, and education need to form a partnership with all people in order to have a major impact on health in this country. Most importantly, *you* must participate in life and take personal responsibility for your health. Make a commitment to be feeling fit.

Appearing in the Videos

Production Agency

Feeling Fit is a production of Media Services Television, Illinois State University, Normal.
Production Staff:
Media Services Television, Illinois State University
John Tannura, Production Manager
Henry Szujewski, Producer/Writer
Jeffrey T. Payne, Producer/Writer
Fred Conner, Production Assistant
Pat Smith, Engineer
Laura DiMascio, Graphic Design
Brad Ochiltree, Graphic Design
Department of Learning Services, WILL-TV, Urbana
Elaine S. Harbison, Director of Learning Services

Donald B. Ardell, PhD

Dr. Ardell is the author of the best-seller, *High Level Awareness and Fourteen Days to A Wellness Lifestyle*, and publisher of the *Ardell Wellness Report*. Dr. Ardell is a consultant and designer of corporate wellness centers throughout the United States. His professional expertise, energy, lifestyle, and personal commitments to wellness have been significant factors contributing to the current level of wellness in the United States.

Richard Bellingham, EdD

Dr. Bellingham is President of Possibilities, Inc., located in Basking Ridge, New Jersey. For the last fifteen years he has consulted on culture change programs for several of the Fortune 500 firms. Dr. Bellingham was senior partner with the Institute for Human Resource Development and has been published in the leading psychological and training journals. He has been the keynote speaker for several regional and national conferences on culture change and health promotion.

Michael Brewer, MD
Dr. Brewer is an Assistant Professor at the Southern Illinois University School of Medicine. He serves as the Associate Resident Director of the Department of Family Practice. He has been actively involved in research related to health promotion and disease prevention.

Margaret Chesney, PhD
Dr. Chesney is Director of the Department of Behavioral Medicine at the Stanford University Research Institute. She is principal investigator for a number of grants from the National Institute of Mental Health and the National Heart, Lung, and Blood Institute that concern a wide range of topics—behavioral risk factors, stress and coping, and women's health in the work environment.

Ronald J. Cook, PhD
Dr. Cook is the Manager of Employee Health Education and Physical Fitness at Sentry Insurance Company in Stevens Point, Wisconsin. Sentry operates the nation's leading corporate fitness programs. Dr. Cook also presents speeches concerning wellness promotion strategies and health in the workplace.

David G. Danskin, PhD
Dr. Danskin is Director of the Counseling Center at Kansas State University. He is a frequent talk-show guest and has appeared on "Good Morning America." His book *Quicki-Mini Stress Management Strategies for Work, Home, Leisure* was the basis for articles in *U.S.A. Today* and *Glamour*.

Mary Jane Darga, RD, MPH
Ms. Darga is Nutrition Specialist at the University of Michigan Medical Center. She works with the American Heart Association preparing such workshops as Cooking for a Healthy Heart.

Michael P. Davies, PhD
Dr. Davies is a Professor of Psychology and the Coordinator of Wellness at St. Louis Community College, Meremac. He is also President of Personal Stress Management, Inc. Dr. Davies conducts stress management and wellness workshops and seminars and is currently investigating biofeedback, relaxation, self-hypnosis, and communication as means of reducing stress.

Harry P. DuVal, PhD
Dr. DuVal is the Director of the University of Georgia at Athens Fitness Center and an Assistant Professor of Physical Education. He has directed the Cardiac Rehabilitation Program of the La Crosse Exercise Program at the University of Wisconsin, La Crosse, and he has conducted research and presentations on community and personal wellness, adult fitness, and cardiac rehabilitation.

David C. Eaton, PhD
Dr. Eaton is Associate Professor of Sociology and Coordinator of Gerontology Programs at Illinois State University, Normal. He has conducted workshops on life planning and church ministries with older persons. His research interests have included a study of children's attitudes toward aging, and economic behavior and consumer choices of older women.

Connie Horton, RN
Ms. Horton has developed support groups for individuals with eating disorders—anorexia nervosa and bulimia. She works with school and community groups in helping people to understand the psychological aspects of eating.

Jane P. Jones, PhD
Dr. Jones is the Acting Director of the National Wellness Institute at the University of Wisconsin, Stevens Point. She has worked as a counselor with individuals and groups from preschool children to adults and has spoken widely on such topics as making life changes, personal well-

ness and health promotion, reducing hypertension, and managing stress. Her writings on these topics can be found in *Life Skills for Human Services Professions* by Gazda, *Human Relations Development* by Gazda, and *Wellness Promotion Strategies* by Opatz.

Sandy Kammermann, MS
Ms. Kammermann is the Wellness Center Manager for the Carle Clinic Association in Urbana, Illinois. She teaches courses in weight control, self-care, and smoking cessation. Additional responsibilities include the marketing of health promotion programs and public relations work with a variety of community advisory committees.

Richard Keelor, PhD
Dr. Keelor is President of Living Well, a Houston-based firm that develops wellness programs for business. He has served as Director of Federal/State Relations for the President's Council on Physical Fitness and Sports. He has appeared in numerous motion pictures about health and fitness.

Susan Kern, PhD
Dr. Kern is Assistant to the President at Illinois State University, Normal. She is a nationally known leader in the area of housing equipment. She is coauthor of *Savvy Consumer* and has a patent on the bi-radiant oven. She has presented numerous workshops on consumerism and women's issues and has served in an advisory capacity for a number of wellness organizations.

Frances Moore Lappe, Honorary Doctorate
Ms. Lappe is an author, a lecturer, and cofounder of the Institute for Food and Development Policy. This not-for-profit institute is internationally recognized for addressing the political and economic causes of world hunger and demonstrating how ordinary citizens can help to end hunger. Coauthor of several publications, Ms. Lappe is best known for her best-selling classic, *Diet for a Small Planet*, and also the *Tenth Anniversary Edition of Diet for a Small Planet*.

Carol A. Lienhard, MS
Ms. Lienhard is the Wellness Coordinator for thirty-five senior centers and sites for the Baltimore County Department of Aging. She has also served as a Nutrition Education Specialist with special expertise in nutrition for the elderly. Ms. Lienhard regularly writes nutrition features for *Senior Digest* newspaper and the column "Food for Thought," and has appeared in televised programs on nutrition for seniors. She also serves as Cochair of the Nutrition Advisory Council of the Maryland State Office of Aging.

Anne Nadakavukaren, MS
Ms. Nadakavukaren is a member of the Health Science Department at Illinois State University. She teaches courses in environmental health and has published a textbook, *Man and Environment*. She is a frequent speaker on environmental issues.

Ann E. Nolte, PhD
Dr. Nolte is Professor of Health Education at Illinois State University, Normal. She is author or coauthor of forty-five books and thirty-one articles. She served as a consultant to President Nixon's Committee on Health Education. She has received many awards for her outstanding contributions to the field of health education.

Susan J. Norris, BS
Ms. Norris is a home economist with the St. Louis District Dairy Council. She has conducted numerous workshops for health professionals and consumer organizations on the prevention and treatment of osteoporosis. She has served as Project Director with the Illinois State Council on Nutrition.

Michael P. O'Donnell, MBA, MPH

Mr. O'Donnell is the Director of Health Promotions Services, Community Health Education at William Beaumont Hospital in San Jose, California. He provides health promotion programs to local employers and also promotes wellness and fitness through community groups. His publications include *Health Promotion in the Workplace* and *Design of Workplace Health Promotion Programs*.

Joseph P. Opatz, PhD

Dr. Opatz is Director of Health Promotion at St. Cloud Hospital, St. Cloud, Minnesota. He has been instrumental in establishing the National Wellness Institute at the University of Wisconsin-Stevens Point. This institute is nationally recognized as a prime source of educational material, workshops, and conferences in the area of wellness and health promotion. A widely known consultant, he has authored *A Primer of Health Promotion: Creating Healthy Organizational Cultures* and has edited *Wellness Promotion Strategies: Selected Procedures of the Eighth Annual National Wellness Conference*.

Cass Overton, BA

Ms. Overton is the Prevention Coordinator of ADAPTS, an alcohol and drug prevention agency in Richmond, Virginia. She has been instrumental in the development of the Richmond Transformational Network, which provides a liaison for persons interested in holistic health, humanistic practice in business, and personal and community growth and direction. Ms. Overton conducts workshops and teaches the art of t'ai chi, an ancient Chinese exercise appropriate for all ages.

George Pfeiffer, MS

Mr. Pfeiffer is Vice-President for the Center for Corporate Health Promotion, Reston, Virginia, immediate past president of the Association for Fitness in Business, and a member of the Corporate Fitness and Recreation's Editorial Advisory Board. He is a nationally known consultant, has authored many articles, and has conducted numerous workshops on wellness at the worksite.

Arlan G. Richardson, PhD

Dr. Richardson is a Professor of Chemistry at Illinois State University. His work in dietary restriction and longevity is internationally known. He has authored over eighty publications and has received over four hundred thousand dollars in grants from the National Institute of Health.

Jane K. Seiler, MA

Ms. Seiler is the Community Fitness and Wellness Director for the Akron Area YMCA. She has been active in promoting community wellness and in working with adult and senior fitness programs as well as adolescent awareness programs.

Al Shepston, BS

Mr. Shepston serves as the host of *Feeling Fit*. He is the program manager of TeleCable in Bloomington-Normal, Illinois. He has been in television broadcasting for fifteen years and has produced promotional materials for Country Companies and General Electric. He is a distance runner and promoter of the *Feeling Fit* lifestyle.

Bernard Siegel, MD, FACS

Dr. Siegel is a surgeon in private practice and Assistant Clinical Professor of Surgery at the Yale University School of Medicine. In 1978 he originated the Exceptional Cancer Patient group therapy, which works with patients' images and drawings. He has written many articles, is currently writing a book (*Love, Medicine, Miracles*), and has appeared on numerous television and radio programs.

Mark M. Tager, MD
Dr. Tager is President of Great Performance, Inc., a Chicago-based consulting firm. A national leader in the field of health promotion, Dr. Tager has authored several books and produced more than a dozen educational videotapes. He is coauthor (with Marjorie Blanchard, PhD) of *Working Well: Managing for Health and High Performance*. He conducts over one hundred educational seminars each year for leaders in business and industry, education, and health care.

Arthur Weltman, PhD
Dr. Weltman, an exercise physiologist, is Health and Physical Education Program Area Director at the University of Virginia. He has worked with the Olympic Committee in the development of weight-training programs for children. He has an extensive background in research and writing and is a nationally known consultant in the areas of fitness and nutrition. His book *Fitness and Nutrition* will soon be available.

Holly Willmann, RD
Ms. Willmann, a registered dietician, develops health promotion programs for Carle Clinic in Urbana, Illinois. She has conducted numerous nutrition education workshops and has helped many people achieve their ideal weight.